Alkaline Diet Cookbook

Complete Guide with Meal Plan and Delicious Recipes to Naturally Rebalance Your pH, Prevent Inflammation and Lose weight. Eat Well to Restore Your Health and Live Longer

By Susan Kellery

TABLE OF CONTENTS

INTRODUCTION

The alkaline diet favours the intake of "alkaline foods" - such as vegetables, fresh fruit, fruit juices, tubers, nuts, and legumes - limiting "acidic foods" such as cereals, meat and cheese; alcohol, cola-type carbonated drinks, and very salty foods are also not recommended.

The alkaline diet is based on the consideration that a diet rich in acidic foods ends up disturbing the acid-base balance of the organism, promoting the loss of essential minerals, such as calcium and magnesium contained in bones.

Such alterations would favour the appearance of mild chronic acidosis, which in turn would be a predisposing factor for certain diseases and for a sense of general malaise.

The alkaline diet recommends to consume every day 70-80% of alkaline foods and 20-30% of acidic foods.

This food model is much closer to that followed by man until the discovery of agriculture than the current one.

CHAPTER ONE: What is the alkaline diet

The Alkaline Diet uses the power of some foods of plant origin with strong anti-inflammatory qualities to promote better health but also to promote weight loss.

The theory behind the alkaline diet consists in dividing the different foods into acidic or alkaline, taking as a reference point the pH scale ranging from 0 to 14.

If the value of the single food is lower than 7, we are in the presence of an acidic food, if higher, than an alkaline food.

It is therefore believed that certain foods, such as meat, wheat, refined sugar and processed foods, are responsible for our body producing acids, which is bad for our health.

Foods rich in sugar and fat increase slightly the acidity of the blood and this promotes inflammation within our body. In response, the body is forced to filter minerals from the bones and organs to restore the correct pH value which is 7.4.

Choosing instead of putting alkaline foods on the table would be a powerful tool that we have in our hands to prevent and combat certain diseases.

Many people who have experienced this style of eating are actually convinced that it is a useful tool to enjoy good health and can also help you to increase your dose of energy.
But what would be the benefits of this diet?

Benefits of the Alkaline Diet

- The advantages of following an alkaline diet would be especially 3:
- **Lose weight**: this type of diet mainly using foods that belong to the plant world and avoiding animal fats can help in weight loss
- **Improve health**: those who follow this diet are convinced that it can be useful especially in the prevention and treatment of inflammation, arthritis and tumors.
  - **Get more energy**: thanks to a diet rich in vitamins and minerals you have the opportunity to see your energy increase in a short time during the various activities carried out every day.

What is acid-alkaline pH

In comparison with other traditional, commercialized diets, the acid-alkaline diet is very new to the public. It recommends a food program rich in fresh fruit and vegetables, roots, nuts, and legumes to sustain and balance body pH.

While the acidity of fish, meat, milk, and salt is created and thus increased in the body, fresh fruits and vegetables are reduced.

Understanding the pH Balance

The pH refers to the alkaline-acid ratio in our body. The pH scale ranges from 0 to 14, and 7 is considered to be neutral.

Anything lower than 7 is considered to be acidic, and anything above 7.1 is considered to be alkaline (also referred to as base).

Once the food we consume has been digested, absorbed, and metabolized, it either releases an acid or a base into our bloodstream. The primary function of alkaline in our system is to neutralize any excess acids and eliminate them from our body.

A body's average pH level is between 7.35 and 7.45 (leaning towards alkaline). Those who support the acid-alkaline diet believe that a diet high in acidic foods upsets the balance, which, in turn, facilitates the loss of minerals essential to us, such as: magnesium, potassium, calcium, and sodium.

If our bodies cannot adequately neutralize the acid, a condition called acidosis can develop. High levels of acid penetrate the body's tissues and can no longer be neutralized. It is thought that acidosis is the one thing that all diseases have in common. Therefore, many doctors believe that the acid-alkaline diet is a healthy regime as it helps maintain the proper PH balance.

How to determine when a foodstuff is acidic?

The acidity of a food is not measured in the fresh state, but on the ashes (minerals) that remain after combustion. These inorganic substances, therefore not metabolizable, can behave as acids or bases, and participate in the maintenance of the normal organic pH.

The lemon, for example, has a very low pH, linked to the abundant presence of citric acid; it is however considered an alkaline food because its acidic components are organic and as such are easily metabolized by the body and eliminated by breathing, while the basic inorganic ones remain longer.

The elements that cause the formation of acids, decreasing the urinary pH, are sulphur, phosphorus and chlorine, while foods rich in sodium, potassium, magnesium and calcium are considered alkaline.

Pral - Potential Renal Acid Load

An index widely used to evaluate the acidifying or alkalizing characteristics of a food is the so-called PRAL (Potential Renal Acid Load).

- foods with negative PRAL (PRAL -) are potentially alkalizing (e.g. vegetables and fruits)
- Foods with positive PRAL (PRAL +) have an acidifying effect (e.g. meat, dairy products, fish and egg yolk).

What is alkaline water

With a pH above 7, alkaline water contains minerals capable of treating the body's acidic organic waste and maintaining a balanced pH in the blood as well as in the body.

As a result, an organism under stress, an acidic diet, and water can acidify and become less resistant to diseases and viruses.

Drinking alkaline water can be a simple gesture, accessible to all and with many virtues to our general health, thanks to its antioxidant properties that protect the body's cells from premature aging due to free radicals. So which alkaline water to choose from and how to alkalize your own tap water?

You should have heard more than once about the healthy properties of alkaline water and its many benefits. Despite not being scientifically proven, there is a lot of information about it, which maintains that it can help delay the aging process, balance the body's pH level and prevent diseases such as bronchial asthma, neuralgia, dermatitis, and others. To measures how acidic or alkaline a substance is on a scale of 0 to 14, with 7 being a neutral point, the alkaline water pH level (hydrogen potential) is more than 7.

It helps to eliminate acids from the body as well as being a natural antioxidant.

Benefits of alkaline water

In addition to balancing the body's pH, consuming alkaline water improves many other aspects of our health, for example, it helps to eliminate toxins from the body, preventing gastrointestinal diseases, constipation, back pain, it prevents the accumulation of free radicals in the body, high cholesterol, neuralgia, among others. It promotes proper digestion, neutralizes gastric acidity, to name a few benefits. It also improves blood circulation and improve the supply of oxygen throughout the body.

Many studies reveal that alkaline water can help prevent premature aging, because by eliminating toxins from the body, it promotes oxygenation of the cells, regenerating them, thus keeping the skin hydrated and elastic.

Almost all diets recommend drinking plenty of water during the day to detoxify the body, they recommend drinking an average of 8 glasses of water per day, according to the age and sex of people, following a healthy and balanced diet rich in fruits and vegetables.

Alkaline water naturally eliminates acids in the body and significantly aids in weight loss because it reduces fat storage. A body with a healthy alkalinity level loses weight more quickly than a body with a high acidity level, all this added to a properly balanced diet.

Also, drinking alkaline water improves the immune system as it neutralizes free radicals and helps cleanse the body of toxins. Therefore, the benefits of alkaline water are vital for long-term health.

Alkaline water is beneficial to your health by neutralizing acids and removing toxins from your body. Tap water usually has a pH value of 7 and is neutral. Alkaline water has a pH range of 7.2 to 9, which is good for the body. The pH value describes the acidity or alkalinity of the water sample. If your body is overly acidic, there is a lack of oxygen in your body cells, and you will not be healthy. When your body is alkaline, and enough minerals are taken from food and drink to remain alkaline, your blood will function normally. To stay healthy it is important to provide oxygen to the body cells and removing all acidic waste from the body.

Too much acid in your body weakens your immune system and can cause several disorders. On the contrary, if your body is basic, it's going to work much better. Alkaline water acts to neutralize the acids present in the body and to remove toxic, acidic waste.

How to get alkaline water

There are different ways to get Alkaline water. It can be

bought packaged in self-service or health food stores. Although it can also be obtained through water purifiers, whose filter system retains sediments and bacteria, providing water with a high quantity of minerals like Sodium, Calcium, Magnesium, and Potassium.

- By installing a Water Purifier and Alkalizer in the tank, this much purer and healthier resource is obtained quickly, 24 hours a day, since you just need to open the tap. It retains 99% of bacteria, improving the quality and taste of water, as it eliminates the taste of chlorine.

Another way to get it is at home. One option is to alkalinize the water by boiling it for 5 minutes; in this way, it will increase its pH to an ideal 8.4 to alkalinize your body.

You can also add half a tablespoon of baking soda to a glass of water. The pH will rise to 7.9 is the degree required to make it alkaline.

- Use sodium bicarbonate. Add 6 g of sodium bicarbonate per 250 ml of water. Bicarbonate has a high alkaline percentage, and when mixed with water, it increases its alkaline properties. Shake the solution (if using a closed container) or Mix (in a glass) vigorously to dissolve the bicarbonate evenly in water. If you follow a diet low in sodium, do not add baking soda to water. Baking soda is high in sodium.
- Use the lemons. Lemons are an anionic food so when you drink water added with lemon juice, your body reacts to its properties by alkalizing the water ingested.Fill a large jug (2 liters) with clean water, better if filtered. If you do not have a suitable filter, you can use normal tap water.Cut a lemon into eight

segments. Dip the segments in water without squeezing.

Cover the carafe and leave the water to rest for 8 hours. 12 hours at room temperature.You might add a pinch of pink Himalayan sea salt. Adding salt mineralizes the alkaline water.

- Add a few drops of concentrated alkaline pH. pH drops contain strong alkaline minerals and have a high concentration. Search the product online and follow the instructions on the packaging to determine the amount of drops to be added to the water. Keep in mind that although the pH drops increase the alkalinity of your water, they do not filter any substance, the fluorine or calcium that may be present in the tap water will therefore continue to remain in your water.

- Buy a water ionizer. Water ionizers are very practical and can be applied to the tap. The water is electrically enhanced (ionized) because it flows through positively and negatively charged ionizer electrodes. The process separates the water into alkaline water and acidic water. Alkaline water makes up about 70% of the water produced and can be drunk.

  Don't just throw acid water. Acid water is able to kill multiple species of bacteria.

- Buy an ionizing filter. It is an easily transportable filter and cheaper than an electric ionizer, which acts similarly to a normal water filter. Pour the water through the filter and wait a few minutes. During this time the water will flow through a series of filters, and then move into a basin of alkalizing minerals. These filters are sometimes available in shops for specialized kitchen tools.

- Buy a reverse osmosis filter. This type of filter is known as hyperfilter, and uses a special very fine membrane for filtering. The sensitivity of the filter allows to retain a greater number of elements than a normal filter, a factor that determines a better alkalinization of the water. Filters of this kind can be purchased in hardware, plumbing or DIY shops, and are often available alongside normal water filters.

- Use a regular water distiller and add concentrated alkaline pH drops. The process of distillation of water purifies its composition, eliminating the bacteria through the increase in temperature, until it reaches boiling. This tool can make your home water slightly more alkaline, although its main task is to purify it by removing the toxins. It is an instrument sold in different measures, and at different prices. You can buy one at any store that specializes in kitchen products.

The amount of water obtained at the end of the processes described will be lower than that used initially. This will happen for any alkalinization method adopted. In the case of reverse osmosis, at least 3 litres of tap water will be required to obtain 1 litre of pure water. Keep the pH level under control for the duration of the alkalinization process, use the appropriate control tools. You will find out which is the most effective method for your water type.

Important: Do not add more bicarbonate to the water than indicated. You may experience physical problems.

Ionized water is rich in antioxidants, and is free from bacteria and other organic substances like chlorine, fluorine, and some metals present in tap water.

It also contains an oxygen atoms and retains healthy minerals.

From the chemical point of view, alkaline water owes its therapeutic capacity to the potential of oxidation-reduction or ORP. This indicator describes the ability of a molecule, ion or compound to transfer electrons (oxidizing - positive ORP), or to receive electrons (shrinking, becoming an antioxidant - negative ORP). In short, thanks to its predominantly alkalizing electrolytes such as calcium, potassium silicate, magnesium and bicarbonate, alkaline water should have a very powerful antioxidant function.

Ionized water protects the body against oxidative damage to protein RNA and DNA.

Alkaline water allows the body to fight aging and other degenerative diseases. Because alkaline water is more readily absorbed by your body cells, it eliminates acid leakage inside the body, and it is less vulnerable to gout, cancer, diabetes, osteoporosis, high blood pressure, and heart disease.

High pH water causes the belly to produce more hydrochloric acid that produces more bicarbonate to the bloodstream. The bicarbonate and the alkaline content in the bloodstream decrease with aging, and the body can not neutralize acids. Increased acidity induces cholesterol, uric acid, kidney stones, and so on. Alkaline ionized water also replenishes calcium deficiency, prevents degradation of bone, and avoids kidney disruption. The alkaline water thus helps the immune system in a variety of ways.

Alkaline Foods and Immune System

Many diseases can develop when a body is in an acidic state. For example, cancer cells will thrive in an acidic environment, and disease can proliferate in such a state. Another common problem that can develop is osteoporosis because when a body is acidic, it is missing sufficient calcium, which is an alkalizing mineral. So clearly, being in an acidic state can contribute to poor health and the onset of various disease conditions. A body that is alkaline has the ability to regenerate more quickly and remove excess toxins more efficiently than an acidic body.

Human beings were truly meant to consume a more alkaline diet, and prior to only the past few recent decades, has man eaten such an acidic diet. Traditionally we have eaten predominantly whole fresh foods, including an abundance of fruits and vegetables. An unfortunate trend in our modern society has been to consume large amounts of processed foods that have contributed to the increase in diseases that proliferate today.

There are many wonderful foods that you can choose from that are alkaline and can help your health and vitality. Raw foods, of course, such as fresh fruits and vegetables are among the most alkaline foods you can consume. In this whole state, you are supplying your body with vital nutrients and enzymes that will nourish your cells and help strengthen your immune system, protecting you from degenerative disease development. Some other top alkalinizing foods include; fresh fruits and vegetables, raw nuts and seeds, sprouted grains, and plenty of fresh, clean water. Try to limit your intake of processed foods, artificial sweeteners, dairy products, and eat meat proteins in moderation. A simple and very effective way to increase your alkalinity is to add a green drink to your daily diet. You can choose from many high-quality products on the market.

CHAPTER TWO: What Are Acidic Foods?

What are foods with acidity? Acidic foods are products that decrease the pH of the body to the acid state. The pH scale has a range from 0 and 14, with 7 being the median balance in a given substance between acid and alkaline existence. The majority of the functions of the human body have a pH balance of 7.4. Cancer can develop when the body sinks into the acidic territory. If it grows past 7.4, cancer will fall asleep and may even die.

Which are Acidic Food Types?

Acidic products are found in a wide variety. Food, milk products, and beer are three common acid offenders. Such products can quickly increase the body's acid content and lead to poor health and a ready breeding ground for cancerous growth as a whole. Although an acid condition in the body delays cancerous development, it does not stop it generally. It is also considered a good probability that an alkaline pH-level body is unable to cause cancer.

What about Protein?

Animal protein, dairy products, and other foods are very healthy to eat at sufficient portions from a strictly nutritional standpoint. Nevertheless, they increase the acidity of foods, which can affect the body's pH level. If consumed with caution when using more alkaline ingredients, the pH balance should usually stay at normal levels. Adjust this diet a bit more, and depending on the change, the risk of developing cancer is either increased or lower.

Why unhealthy is a diet with high acidity?

A highly acidic diet is rich in foods like animal protein and many other processed caloric items. Many of those foods can cause severe health problems without adequate portion control without even considering the quality of their acids. Therefore, a high acid diet reduces the amount of oxygen that can enter the cells and allows internal acids, such as lactic acid, to build up in cells. This is usually why cancers develop if the cause is not certain external factors. Inhalation of asbestos is an example of an indirect cancer cause that has little to do with the acid content of food, although all cancers seem to need a slightly acidic or balanced body.

Acid-based diets lead to waste materials and various free radicals that develop cancer within the body. The alkaline diet can be used to purify free radicals and to improve their oxygen content in cancer cells, killing them even as the increased blood flow and oxygen invigorate normal healthy tissues.

Why can I test the balance of my pH?

What are acidic foods? and how do I test my pH balance? There are tools that can be used for this purpose called' acid strips' or' pH strips.' The individual's saliva is usually used as the body fluid is easy to reach and works well in pH balance testing. A balance that indicates a number below 7.4 means that the body is more acidic, while a degree above 7.4 means that the body is more alkaline and normal. 7 is the exact foundation of anything above 7 alkaline and anything under 7 acidic.

The influence of alkaline and acidic foods on our health

The influence of alkaline and acidic foods on our health is determined above all by erroneous dietary habits. This has a negative effect on our health and is directly related to the necessary balance in the pH of our interior terrain.

We will see first what pH is

PH or Hydrogen Potential is a measure of the concentration of hydrogen ions and shows the degree of alkalinity or acidity of a solution. A pH below 7.0 is acidic, while a pH above 7.0 is alkaline. It is known that the pH of human blood should be slightly alkaline and that it should be kept between the values 7.35 to 7, 45 since if they were above or below these figures, the body would become ill or begin to show symptoms of illness. A blood pH of 6.9, which is only slightly acidic, can induce coma and death. Therefore, the body has the so-called Buffer systems to quickly compensate for any deviation in this balance.

Mild Chronic Acidosis

That said, what is important to know is that what we are talking about is not acidosis itself, but mild chronic acidosis. The important problem is not exactly in the blood (which if there is also), but in our liquids, in our extracellular matrix or the Basic System of Pischinger. Studies by Austrian Alfred Pischinger (1966) revealed the significance of the connective system for cellular function. Also known as connective tissue, mesenchyme or extracellular matrix, SBP is responsible for the most elementary basic functions of life: exchange of water, oxygen, electrolytes, acid-alkaline regulation as well as everything related to nonspecific defense systems. It is this "interior terrain" that slowly and chronically loses its "cleanliness" (alkalinity) and "gets dirty," creating mild chronic acidosis.

Having an acidic pH can be due to different reasons; among them, we have an acidic diet, emotional stress, toxic overload, and immune reactions or any process that deprives the cells of oxygen and other nutrients, etc. If this is so, then the body will attempt to compensate for the acidic pH using alkaline minerals. However, if our diet does not contain enough minerals to compensate for it, there will be an excessive accumulation of acids in our interior terrain.

An acid imbalance can:

- reduce the body's ability to absorb minerals and other nutrients
- reduce energy production in cells
- reduce the ability to repair damaged cells
- reduce the body's ability to detoxify heavy metals
- Allowing tumor cells to grow makes you more susceptible to fatigue and illness.
- Main Cause of Mild Chronic Acidosis

The reason that mild chronic acidosis is so common in our society is the typical Western diet, which is too high in acid due to excessive consumption of animal products such as meat, eggs, and dairy products, refined cereal flours, and too much low in alkaline foods like mostly fresh vegetables. In addition, we receive acidic residues produced by processed foods such as refined cereal flours, white sugar, and acid from beverages such as coffee and soft drinks. We also use too many medications, which are acid generators, and we use artificial chemical sweeteners like NutraSweet, Aspartame, and others, which are extreme acid formers.

Acid Dietary Errors

All these problems and dietary errors make our digestion sick and cause or trigger what is surely the largest producer of acids in our system: a diseased colon. It is slowly irritated, inflamed, and hurt for months and years of receiving poor quality food like the ones mentioned above. Once the tissues have been caused by these micro-wounds, they will begin to let small particles and proteins pass without digesting into the bloodstream. This is known as Intestinal Permeability Syndrome. When this occurs, the immune system reacts violently to these unknown particles, causing the so-called "Allergic Reactions".

In addition, the mucoid plaque layers stick to the interior of the tissue and cause poor absorption of electrolytes (water and minerals). And this can be one of the reasons for our mild chronic dehydration, dry skin, and a host of other health problems.

Eating an Alkaline Diet full of alkaline foods

One of the things that we can do simply, cheaply and quickly, so that our interior terrain is not too acidic is to change our diet and lifestyle.

To maintain health, our diet must consist of 60% alkaline foods and 40% acidic foods. But to restore health, our diet must consist of 80% alkaline foods and 20% acidic foods. The latter is the case of most of the population in the countries that we believe to be "developed."

In general, alkaline foods include most fruits, vegetables, peas, beans, lentils, algae, spices, herbs and condiments, seeds, and nuts.

Acidic foods generally include: meat, fish, poultry, eggs, cereals, and legumes.

It should be very clear that we are not trying to classify foods into "bad" and "good" categories. There are no bad foods in their natural form. Alkaline foods or acidic foods are only more useful or less useful, depending on the specific needs at any given time in a certain person.

Using alkaline foods or acidic foods to adjust your pH

This section is for those who want to "adjust" or balance their body's PH. The PH scale is 0 to 14, with the numbers below 7 being acidic (low in oxygen) and the numbers above 7, alkaline. An acidic body is a magnet for the disease. What you eat and drink will have a decisive impact on the PH level in your body. Remember that balance is the key!

Acidosis and Inflammation

Our bodies need to maintain a number of constants, including acidity, to function properly. For example, if the acidity of the blood, its pH, comes out of the range 7.35 and 7.45, there is a risk of discomfort, even death. Without going that far, many health problems are linked to too high acidity. An often unbalanced diet and a sedentary lifestyle mean that many people are faced with chronic acidosis and its series of ailments.

Some symptoms encountered in chronic acidosis

Fatigability, dull/drooping/brittle hair, brittle / split / scratched nails, dry skin, muscle or joint pain, rheumatism, osteoporosis, chilliness, cold extremities, cramp, spasms, lack of energy, difficulty recovering, depressive tendency, irritability, nervousness, emotionality, dental problems, kidney stones, urinary or rectal burns, inflammation of the mucous membranes, lowered immunity, allergies, and others.

How acidosis disrupts the functioning of the body

- By the loss of minerals (used to neutralize acids). The various organs and tissues that provide buffer minerals do so by demineralizing. The bones are the first affected (calcium), but also the nervous system (magnesium). Demineralization can prevent certain reactions from taking place, which can lead, like enzymatic disturbances, to an increase in acid charge. Acidosis promotes osteoporosis by eliminating calcium from the bones, which are used to neutralize the excess of acidity.
- By disrupting the proper functioning of enzymes that need a specific pH to function properly. Thus the acidity can prevent the realization of physiological reactions and, in particular, the production of proteins and hormones. The intermediate stages of certain reactions go through the creation of acidic elements. If following an enzymatic problem, these products remain in the state in the body, there is an increase in acidity.
- By reducing the immune system, for the same reasons as enzymes.
- By promoting the inflammation of the tissues by acids or deposits of crystals (the salts resulting from the

buffer system by the basifying minerals), thus causing diseases in "it's" and in "oses." Inflammation of the tissues, in addition to the discomfort felt, weakens the tissues against infections.

- The formation of deposits, blockage of joints, stones, due to the formation of "crystals" during the neutralization of acids. Because an acid linked to a base gives a neutral salt and water, but this neutral salt is not always easily eliminated and remains in the body.

How the body regulates acidity

- PH measures acidity on a scale of 0 (maximum acid) to 14 (maximum alkaline), passing through equilibrium 7 (neutral like water). The more acid an element, the more it contains H + ion.
- In a healthy body, the pH of the blood is between 7.35 and 7.45; that of the skin around 5.2; that of urine between 6.5 and 7.5. If the pH of the skin and urine can vary beyond its values, the blood should not go beyond its limits, at the risk of discomfort, even death.
- The acidity can be regulated in two ways: Either it is eliminated (mainly in the urine and by breathing), or it is neutralized by basic minerals which give neutral salts (buffer systems). The body preferably seeks to eliminate acids, but it does not always have the capacity to eliminate acids quickly enough, it is then that buffer systems come into play. If these allow the return to a normal acid-base balance, they cause demineralization.

How to get off acid from your body

1. Reduce consumption of animal products

Once metabolized, proteins of animal origin secrete acid waste in the body, including uric acid, sulfuric acid, or phosphoric acid, which are difficult to eliminate, which unbalances the acidity levels of the organism. Red meats, cheeses, and cold meats, in particular, are among the most acidifying foods for the human body. So, unless they come from organic farming, be sure to reduce your consumption of meats, but also of fish, especially in the evening.

2. Multiply your consumption of foods rich in fiber

Fiber is ideal for reducing acidity levels in the body. So be sure to consume it regularly. These are naturally present in cereals, such as oat, flax, barley seeds, or even wheat germ. Spices, such as cayenne pepper, oilseeds, seaweed, or fruits and vegetables, are also excellent sources of fiber. You can also quite consume them in infusion, in particular the seeds of flax.

3. Prepare infusions

Most remineralizing plants are known for their alkalizing properties. Among them, nettle, flowering oats, bamboo, raspberry, or even horsetail are preferred infusions. Regarding tea, choose green or white tea rather than black tea, which is a little more acidifying.

4. Stay well hydrated, in all circumstances

Not only is water essential for the proper functioning of the human body, but it is also a particularly alkalizing element. Make sure you consume enough water throughout the day to avoid dehydration problems.

You can consume water in all its forms. Lemon water, for example, is excellent; drink every morning on an empty stomach a glass of warm water with a lemon. If citric acid is an acid, once metabolized, it has great alkalizing properties. For a more alkaline body, you can also add a spoon of baking soda.

5. Reduce consumption of industrial food

The processed foods, and thus processed, are particularly discouraged, whether for their acidifying properties, but also for their misdeeds on health. Practical, attractive, and quick to prepare, they certainly save precious time. But at what cost? Packed with preservatives, texturing agents, and harmful compounds, ready meals, and other industrial sauces facilitate acidification of the body. Choose homemade dishes made from natural ingredients.

6. Reduce your consumption of refined foods, especially white flour

In the same way, as for the processed foods mentioned above, refined foods are to be avoided. Indeed, white flours, like white sugar and table salt, undergo industrial cleaning and bleaching processes, which make them lose all their nutritional properties. Nutrients, minerals, and fiber are eliminated, which greatly reduces the value of these foods.

7. Consume alkalizing foods

Alkalizing foods will make the body less acidic and, therefore, more alkaline. This is the case with healthy fruits and vegetables, which have many health benefits. Many green vegetables, in particular, are known for their alkalizing properties. Thus, asparagus, cucumber, broccoli, zucchini, artichoke, or even green pepper, are very effective in rebalancing the acid-base balance in the body. You can also consume them as a "green" smoothie.

Choose raw vegetables, which are excellent sources of vitamins, minerals, fiber, and trace elements. Loaded with oxygen, they also have natural enzymes that eliminate accumulated toxins and strengthen the body's natural defenses. They are particularly alkalizing.

Also, be sure to turn to organic fruits and vegetables to avoid overconsumption of pesticides, chemical fertilizers, and other toxins, which promote acidification of the body.

8. Choose the right cosmetic products

Certain treatments or cosmetic products can have harmful effects on your skin and/or hair. So, for your beauty products, choose organic and all-natural brands, which will help you keep your skin/teeth/hair healthy and healthy.

9. Take care of your lifestyle: physical activity and sleep

As we have seen, diet is not the only responsible for disorders linked to acidity levels in the body. Lack of sleep and stress also negatively affect pH. So be sure to sleep an average of 6-

7 hours per night, following a regular rhythm, for a better quality of sleep. This will affect your wellbeing and mood.

Also, practice regular physical activity; sport, whatever it is, is indeed ideal for increasing the secretion of endorphins in the body, hormones of wellbeing, and happiness.

You can also turn to activities designed to reduce stress levels, and therefore maintain the acid-base balance of the human body. It is not for nothing that yoga, and the various meditation techniques, are enjoying increasing success today.

10. Choose your household products with care

Household products can also cause risks to the body's acidity levels. They are true, in general, stuffed with sometimes harmful chemical elements, generally called endocrine disruptors. So carefully check the composition of your cleaning products. Choose products that are 100% natural, and just as effective - if not more - like baking soda, lemon, or white vinegar.

How Stress can cause acid

Acid reflux is often one of the most common complaints, affecting just about everyone at one time or another. Also known as GERD (Gastro-Esophageal Reflux Disease), this is something known to all of us as heartburn. The characteristic symptoms of acid reflux are due to stomach acids entering the esophagus; the name "heartburn" is due to the pain of acid reflux that is usually felt in the center of the chest.

There are several factors that can trigger acid reflux. Many find that they are prone to symptoms after eating certain foods, especially acidic foods such as tomatoes and citrus fruits. Fried food is also believed by many to cause acid reflux. But is it possible that stress causes acid reflux? The general consensus is yes, and few of us have not experienced the symptoms of acid reflux at a time of particularly acute stress. The truth of the matter, however, is a little more complex.

While most people are saying yes if they are asked, "does stress cause reflux of acid? " it does happen that stress simply does not cause reflux of acid in itself. Stress can, however, be a worsening factor that can make acid reflux symptoms appear even worse than they are. We all know how discomfort enhances uncomfortable sensations-and that definitely extends to heartburn.

Some agree that stress can be a factor in acid reflux; one of the reasons we are more likely to heartburn in tense periods is that we all want to consume comfort in response to higher rates of tense. Furthermore, foods to which we prefer to turn for warmth are also known to induce acid reflux. In addition to our heightened vulnerability in times of stress, we are more likely to experience an acid reflux attack, and it can look much worse than otherwise.

Researches have shown that acid reflux symptoms can be improved by calming strategies. If you suffer from a high degree of stress, consider relaxation exercises and exercise to relieve the stress, this can help to reduce acid reflux in away. In such cases, walking is an especially good workout. Maintaining an upright stance is a safe way to avoid stomach acids from penetration and heart pain, so walking in and of itself can be really calming.

You can reduce the intensity and the frequency of the acid reflux symptoms by keeping an eye on what you eat and using stress management techniques. Remember, can stress response induce reflux of acid? Not - but stress can make the acid reflux symptoms even worse than they would otherwise, and it can also cause heartburn in certain situations that people deal with stress.

Metabolism reset and weight loss with the alkaline diet

The intent is to achieve an acid-alkaline balance in food intake. In other words, substitute sugars, flours, and fats for fruits and vegetables.

The consumption of alkaline foods protects us from certain diseases and improves our metabolism by immediately affecting the pH of our body.

PH is the acidity level of the body. It is measured on a scale of 0 to 14. From 0 to 7, it is considered an acidic body and from 7 onwards, alkaline. The objective is to achieve the maximum possible balance, consuming 80% alkaline foods and 20% acids.

With this diet, it is possible to detoxify the body through urine, which will eliminate toxins and protect us from diseases and infections. At the same time, by leaving out greasy or sugar-rich foods, your metabolism will improve, and your weight will decrease.

Food alkaline diet for weight loss

- Vegetables: Broccoli, carrot, green beans, cauliflower, beet, cucumber, peppers, lettuce, onion, garlic, spinach, bean sprouts, tomato, cabbage, asparagus, etc.
- Fruits: Mango, papaya, apricots, apple, grapes, coconut, watermelon, melon, cherry, peach, tangerine, lemon, pear, pineapple, plum, etc.
- Legumes: Lentils
- Nuts: Chestnuts, raisins, hazelnuts, almonds, walnuts, and dates.
- Spices: cayenne, ginger, cinnamon, herbs, curry, parsley, and chili.
- Condiments: Baking soda, mineral water, salt, honey, and apple cider vinegar.
- Drinks: Tea and infusions
- Oils: Olive oil.
- In addition, there is a fundamental food in the alkaline diet to lose weight: lemon. Mixed with baking soda, it helps to balance our body towards the alkaline side.

Stages of the alkaline diet to lose weight

We must start the diet little by little, gradually introducing alkaline foods. These are the phases to follow in the alkaline diet.

Debugging phase: In this first three-week stage, the toxins in our body are eliminated, and we begin to lose weight. We can reduce a kilo of weight a week.

Quick start phase: In the second phase, lasting four weeks, the weight loss is consolidated, and the pH is increasingly balanced. We will drop from 500 to 750 grams a week.

Sustained Advance Phase: Like the previous phase, it also lasts four weeks. Our energy level increases and the weight loss continues constantly. A week it is possible to lose 500 grams.

Consolidation phase : this phase lasts two weeks and allows us to definitively establish our diet plan to maintain the same weight for the rest of our lives.

Alkaline and Acidic foods

Among the absolutely most alkalizing foods there is the grape, in fact often this fruit appears in detoxifying diets.

Other alkaline foods are: beets, turnips, carrots, radishes, cabbages, cauliflower, broccoli, spinach, garlic, lemons, cucumbers, celery, apples, dried figs, bean sprouts, lettuce, avocados and mushrooms. Among the condiments from the alkalizing power there are ginger, chili, curry, sage, rosemary, cumin seeds and fennel seeds. The only alkalizing cereals (or similar grains) are quinoa, millet and amaranth.

In summary, when following an alkaline diet, you should increase the intake of:

Grape

Beets

Turnips

Carrots

Radishes

Cabbage

Cauliflower

Broccoli

Spinach

Garlic

Lemon

Cucumbers

Celery

Apples

figs

bean sprouts

lettuce

avocado

mushrooms

mile

quinoa

amaranth

ginger

chilli

curry

sage

rosemary

fennel seeds

cumin seeds

extra virgin olive oil

linseed oil

walnuts and oilseeds

There are different alkalizing foods but this does not mean that you should always eat those. Even exceeding with the alkalinization of the body can lead to disadvantages. As always, you must know how to use the right means and, if possible, avoid DIY but rely on the advice of an expert who will best calibrate the best diet to be followed on the individual case.

More than foods to avoid, it would be better to talk about foods to limit when you need to alkalize your body.

Foods that contain yeast and sugar, refined, processed, microwave-cooked but also fermented, are considered acidifying. Cereals are almost all acidifying: wheat, spelt, oats, rice, rye, corn, barley and all their derivatives, including bread and pasta. Even some legumes are acidifying among them chickpeas, white beans and lentils. Animal proteins include meat, but also fish such as cod, salmon as well as eggs, milk and cheese. Among the sweeteners to limit there are sugar and honey.

Summarizing the foods to limit are:

Yeasts

Sugar

refined or treated foods

cooked or microwave-heated foods

fermented food

wheat

spelt

oats

rye

rice

corn

barley

bread and pasta

chickpeas

white beans

lentils

flesh

fish

eggs

cheese and milk

honey

As we have already specified the foods listed above are not

necessarily to be eliminated completely, but is important to find the right food balance avoiding the excessive formation of acids within our body.

For example, if you realize that your diet is too unbalanced in favor of acidifying foods you can start to insert more alkalizing foods daily.

Health Benefits of an Alkaline Diet

A person might choose to follow an alkaline diet for many reasons. It is common for people to go on a diet for one specific reason, only to discover many other improvements in their lives as a result. Here you can find some of the health benefits of an alkaline diet that could make it the right choice for you:

Improved Energy Levels

An alkaline diet is known for its boost to the energy level of a human. The typical diet is high in refined foods, added sugar, fat, and food supplements that can drain the individual's level of energy. Such foods are not only difficult for the body to absorb, but they also promote weight gain, which can cause another drain of energy. On the other hand, if you provide your body with the fresh fruits, vegetables, legumes, nuts, and essential oils it needs for good health, your level of energy will possibly increase significantly.

Your body can easier absorb this natural food so that after you have eaten, you won't feel the energy level that is so normal with a fatty and sugar diet. This would also be easier for the internal organs to work properly if you keep the pH alkaline rather than acidic. More stress for your body means higher levels of energy for you.

Resistance to Disease and Illness

Alkaline diets are also the safest way to popularize the risk of getting sick. The body is better able to fight infections if the symptoms of acidity do not also occur. If the pH of the body is preserved to approximately 7.3, all body functions, including cardiovascular, respiratory, and digestive systems, will be able to operate at optimum efficiency.

The foods typically consumed in an alkaline diet are normal, fresh, and nutritious as an additional bonus. Processed foods, most of which acidify, contain food additives and chemicals which can contribute to the body's toxicity. When the body combats toxicity, it becomes more vulnerable to disease. You will increase your overall wellbeing by eliminating these items from your diet.

 A high level of acid in the body can also help to develop other illnesses, such as cancer. By maintaining the pH of the body at a relatively alkaline level, you can avoid these diseases. Most people often experience improved allergy tolerance and fewer breathing issues when transitioning to an alkaline diet. It is partly attributable to the fact that many acid foods often contain mucous foods. Once nasal and pulmonary inflammation is eliminated from the food, it decreases and enhances breathing.

Alkaline diet, Weekly Plan

Those who want to experience the benefits in first person can try to follow the alkaline diet for 7 days.

The alkaline diet allows to eat mainly foods of vegetable origin (although not all foods are actually alkalizing, an example for all is wheat and other cereals considered acidic).

It is essential to know that acid foods should not be completely eliminated from our diet but that the right daily proportion should be the one that sees the introduction of an 80% of alkaline foods and a 20% of acidic foods.

This is an example of a weekly alkaline diet plan. You can ask an expert to draw up one calibrated to your specific needs.

Alkaline 2 weeks Diet Plan

I suggest to start always with a cup of warm water and lemon when wake up.

Day 1

Breakfast: quinoa puffed with vegetable milk and fresh fruit

Snack: a seasonal fruit

Lunch: salad with lettuce, cucumber, avocado and a handful of pistachios

Snack: a handful of toasted nuts or other dried fruit

Dinner: chicken with roast potatoes and salad seasoned with extra virgin olive oil and apple vinegar

Day 2

Breakfast: muesli with vegetable milk and fresh fruit

Lunch: fresh fruitLunch: avocado and lettuce rolls, with red onion plus white bean stew

Snack: a handful of roasted pumpkin seeds

Dinner: roast fish with Brussels sprouts or red peppers (depending on the season). Cucumber salad with olive oil and apple vinegar.

Day 3

Breakfast: red fruit smoothie

Snack: 1 mango

Lunch: rice noodles with vegetables

Snack: a handful of dried apricots

Dinner: zucchini spaghetti with black cabbage pesto

Day 4

Breakfast: oatmeal, coconut milk and almond butter

Snack: a banana

Lunch: avocado salad with chopped cabbage and broccoli, seasoned with mixed vegetable seeds, oil and lemon

Snack: a handful of almondsDinner: roast chicken with baked sweet potatoes and beets

Day 5

Breakfast: fruit smoothieSnack: a fresh fruit

Lunch: quinoa with vegetables

Snack: a handful of dates

Dinner: risotto with mushrooms and almond flakes

Day 6

Breakfast: chia puddingS

Snack: half a cup of blueberries

Lunch: miso soup with fermented tofu

Snack: a handful of macadamia nuts

Dinner: salmon with roasted vegetables

Day 7

Breakfast: porridge with oats and berries

Snack: a seasonal fruit

Lunch: quinoa salad

Snack: a handful of dried fruit of your choice

Dinner: pumpkin cream soup

Day 8

Breakfast: extract of fruit and/or vegetables

Lunch: millet with seasonal vegetables and an apple

Snacks: fresh or dried fruit

Dinner: Grilled or baked fish seasoned with olive oil and raw lemon with vegetables

Day 9

Breakfast: fresh fruit salad

Lunch: amaranth flan with vegetables

Snacks: centrifuged or extract of fruits and vegetables

Dinner: Legume soup with raw extra virgin olive oil with vegetables

Day 10

Breakfast: water and lemon and then extract or fruit or vegetable

Lunch: a quinoa salad with vegetables and seasoned with extra virgin olive oil.

Snacks: raw vegetables or fruit

Dinner: tofu with seasonal vegetables

Day 11

Breakfast: fresh seasonal fruit

Lunch: vegetable and legume soup with croutons

Dinner: vegetable burger with vegetables

Snacks: fresh or dried fruit or green tea

Day 12

Breakfast: juice or fruit and vegetable extract

Lunch: Risotto with asparagus or other seasonal vegetables and mixed salad

Snacks: orange juice or fresh fruit

Dinner: salmon with potatoes

Day 13

Breakfast: seasonal fruit

Lunch: Whole-grain cereal cake with vegetables

Snacks: green tea, fresh or dried fruit

Dinner: chickpea hummus with vegetables and whole wheat bread

Day 14

Breakfast: water and lemon, fruit salad

Lunch: salad with seasonal mixed vegetables, avocado and oilseeds

Snacks: fresh or dried fruit

Dinner: legume meatballs with vegetables

Day 15 (Extra)

Breakfast: soy yogurt and a fruit

Snack: orange juice and fruit

Lunch: a plate of wholemeal pasta (80 grams) seasoned with broccoli sautéed in a pan with garlic and a teaspoon of oil, 50 grams of mixed salad seasoned with a little oil and lemon juice.

Snack: a piece of dark chocolate and a fruit.

Dinner: 100 grams of tofu sautéed in a pan, a plate of raw or cooked seasonal vegetables and a fruit.

CHAPTER THREE: Recipes

ALKALINE BREAKFAST

- Quinoa and Apple -

ingredients for 2 people:
½ cup of quinoa
1 apple
½ lemon
Cinnamon
raisins (optional)

Preparation

Bring the quinoa to the boil and cook for 15 minutes. Then, grate the apple and cook for another 30 seconds, grate the zest of a lemon and squeeze a small lemon to taste. Note: if you want to add raisins, add it just before you put the apple.

- Avocado Breakfast On-the-Go -

ingredients for one person:
Half avocado
¼ of lemon
a handful of sesame seeds Linseed oil
A Clove of garlic
½ tomato

Preparation

Dice the tomato, crush the garlic and empty the avocado with the spoon, keeping the skin intact. Mix everything with lemon and oil and then place it in the empty skin of the avocado, a pinch of Himalayan salt and serve

- Raw Almond Milk -

Ingredients
1 cup of almonds
3 cups of water
1 vanilla pod

Preparation

Place the almonds in water overnight in an airtight container in the refrigerator. Drain the old water and then mix the almonds with new water (3 cups) until they are more or less all nice and smooth. Now filter with a strainer gauze or other. you can store it for about 3 days in the refrigerator.

ALKALINE SALADS

- Powerful salad -

Ingredients for 2 people:
1 can of chickpeas
1 stalk of celery
Small leaves of spinach
Leaves of Roman lettuce
3 tomatoes
3 spring onions
1 red pepper
1 avocado
1 bunch of asparagus
1 lemon juice for seasoning
olives oil

Preparation

Chop and mix all the ingredients in a large bowl, allowing the avocado to blend with the salad

- Tofu Salad with Fruits -

100 grams of tofu

50 grams mixed salad

1 kiwi

1 tablespoon corn

1 carrot

5 green olives pitted

1 tablespoon mixed seeds (pumpkin, flax, sunflower, sesame)

1 teaspoon extra virgin olive oil

1 pinch of salt

orange juice

1/2 teaspoon dried mixed aromatic herbs

Preparation

Prepare an emulsion with orange juice, oil, salt and aromatic herbs. Wash and cut the vegetables and fruits, then mix all the ingredients in a salad bowl and season.

It is an ideal single dish to bring to work, for a balanced and tasty meal but simple and quick to prepare.

ALKALINE SOUPS

- Tunisian soup of chickpea -

Ingredients for 4 people:
350g dried chickpeas, soaked in cold water for one night and drained
10 cloves of garlic, cut into very thin pieces
2 and 1/2 litres of ionised alkaline water
8 tablespoons extra virgin olive oil
2 carrots, cut julienne
5 celery stalks, cut into thin slices
2 finely chopped onions
1 teaspoon ground cumin
1 teaspoon ground coriander
4 tablespoons chopped coriander
Lemon juice
Himalayan salt crystal
black pepper

Preparation

Heat half the olive oil over at low heat in a large pot. Add the garlic and steam for about two minutes. Add chickpeas, water, cumin and coriander. Boil all ingredients. Reduce heat and boil for about 2 1/2 hours. Meanwhile heat the remaining oil in a pan, add the carrots, onions and celery. Mix during cooking time. Add the vegetables to the soup and mix well. Take about half of the broth and make a puree in a mixer. Add the puree to the soup and mix well. Give flavor to the soup with salt, pepper and lemon juice. Serve the soup and garnish with fresh coriander.

- Leek and asparagus soup -

Ingredients for 4 people
800g of green asparagus
3 leeks, peeled and chopped
1/2 lemon
2 tablespoons olive oil
4 cups vegetable broth
Himalayan salt crystal
Freshly ground pepper

Preparation

Cut the asparagus. Set the tips of the asparagus aside because they will be used later. Chop the asparagus stalks. Add oil in a large pan and brown the leeks for about 10-15 minutes until they begin to soften. Add the broth and cut the asparagus stalks into small pieces and cook with a lid for about 25 minutes. Place the soup in a kitchen robot and mix ore use a hand blender. Season the soup to taste, add the asparagus tips and bring the soup back to the boil. Cook the soup for other 5 minutes. Add the fresh lemon juice.

- Soup for muscle strength -

Ingredient for 4-6 people
1 avocado
1 cup of water or vegetable broth
2 cucumbers
1 cup raw spinach
2 onions
1 garlic
1/2 red pepper

Sea salt
Spices (garam masala, curry, etc.)

Preparation

In a blender, add the avocado and half the water or broth. Make a purée, then add the rest of the ingredients (except green mint leaves), one at a time, stir and dilute with the remaining water if desired. Season to taste with salt and spices and lemon juice. This soup can be served hot or cold.

- Vegetable soup -

Ingredients
250 grams of seasonal vegetables per person
40 grams of dried legumes per person
1 potato
60 grams of brown rice per person
1 onion, a celery stalk, a carrot and a clove of garlic
1 tablespoon of oil
Aromatic herbs (bay leaves, sage, rosemary, basil)
salt

Preparation:

Clean and cut vegetables.
Fry together onion, celery, carrot and garlic and sauté for a few minutes in olive oil. Add potato and legumes previously soaked, rice and cover with water. Add the herbs and cook for about half an hour on low heat; Then add the rest of the vegetables and complete cooking for another thirty minutes.

ALKALINE SHAKES

- Vegetable Juice to Rebuild Blood -

This juice is absolutely full of chlorophyll and is incredibly highly alkaline.

Ingredients for 2 people:
1 cucumber
2 handfuls of large spinach
1 handful of parsley
1 stalk of celery
Handful of Kale

Preparation

wash all the ingredients, chop coarsely and make the juice! To give a fruitier flavor squeeze fresh lime or lemon at the end.

- Avocado Alkaline Power Shake -

Ingredients for 2 people:

1 cucumber

2 tomatoes

1 avocado

1 handful of spinach leaves

1 lime

½ red pepper

½ teaspoon of vegetable broth

Preparation

Wash all ingredients thoroughly and then chop cucumber, tomato, bell pepper and avocado. Dissolve the vegetable broth in a small amount (50 ml) of warm water. Place the avocado and broth in the blender and stir until it becomes a cream. Then, add the ingredients with high water content in a blender and blend until it becomes increasingly liquid. Finally, add the spinach and lime until all the ingredients are well mixed. Serve in a tall glass.

- Green Salad Alkaline Shake -

Ingredients for a person:

1 avocado

1 green pepper

1 handful of salad leaves (for example Roman or iceberg)

1/2 cucumber

1 tomato

1/2 lemon juice

1 handful of flaxseed

Preparation

Cut into pieces cucumber, tomato, avocado salad leaves and bell pepper.

Mix all the ingredients with the highest setting until everything is well mixed together.

- Protein shake to increase pH -

ingredients

1 avocado, peeled and crushed

1 lime, peeled and cut in half

1 cucumber, roughly chopped

Tofu from half to one cube

Soy milk - look for sugar-free milk (add according to your own taste / desired consistency)

1-2 large handfuls of fresh leaves of raw spinach

Ice at will (if your blender is able to handle ice)

Preparation

Peel the avocado and lime and wash the cucumber thoroughly. Then put all the ingredients in a blender and blend everything.

- Garlic tea and Ginger Tonic -

Ingredients

4 cloves garlic, chopped

4 pieces of grated ginger root

1 lemon juice

a pinch of cayenne pepper

500ml of IONIZED ALKALINE water.

Preparation

Prepare all the ingredients and put them on a large cup.

Cover with freshly boiled water and leave to infuse for 15-20 minutes. Filter and drink.

- Lemon-lime -

Ingredients for one person

1 avocado

1/2 cucumber

1 lime (peeled)

2 lemons (juice)

1 coconut

1 teaspoon stevia

6 ice cubes

Preparation

Insert the ingredients into the blender. Low-speed mixture to start. As soon as it becomes liquid blend at high speed until it becomes smooth and fluffy.

- Vegetable curry -

Ingredients for 4-6 people

1 chopped onion
1 bay leaf
1 green chili pepper
1 clove of chopped garlic
1 piece of ginger, grated
1/4 teaspoon turmeric
Sea salt to give flavor
1 lb diced carrots
1/2 cauliflower cut into florets
1 cup green peas
1 teaspoon of coriander
1 teaspoon cumin
1 cup hot water

Preparation

Sauté onion. Add bay leaf, chilli pepper, garlic, ginger, turmeric and salt. Add the carrots and fry slightly.

Add the other ingredients. Cook gently over medium heat until the vegetables are tender.

Tips for an alkaline lifestyle

Our diet has changed over the last 50 to 60 years. We're no longer eating a natural diet from a garden or a local farm. Canned, frozen, packaged, processed, and fast food is now readily available and has increased in our diet since the 1950s. Because of our busy and fast-paced life, many people eat these "convenience" foods in their daily diet. During this time, diseases are also on the increase, and new diseases are on the rise every year.

Many people think that diet is something they're doing to lose weight or keep a disease in check, such as heart disease or diabetes. Diet is simply eating and drinking the right foods that provide the body with optimum nutrition. What you put in your mouth is a choice that you make, and when your choices make you suffer, as in poor health, you can change those choices and change the outcome that you experience.

Food is needed to feed the cells in your body and keep them healthy. Many people, however, have abused the true meaning of why they eat food. They eat for social and emotional reasons, because of food addiction and cravings. They eat too much of the wrong kind of food that causes excess weight and poor health. The right type of protein, carbohydrate, and fat, together with the right balance of each meal, will promote better health and weight loss.

What you eat is just a part of maintaining good health. Negative thoughts, physical and emotional stress, toxins in your home, and the surrounding environment can also contribute to illness, illness, and aging. Poor choices lead to problems. Changing the way you eat, think, and live can help you get back to homeostasis. You can start with the first step of eating an alkaline diet.

tips for alkalinizing your body

1. Correct your diet

Intake fo green leafy vegetables in your diet, such as spinach, broccoli, arugula, lettuce, also tomatoes, cucumbers, legumes such as chickpeas and lentils, seeds such as walnuts, almonds, hazelnuts, lemon, lime, cereals such as quinoa. Ideally, our foods should be 80% alkaline and 20% acidic to maintain a balance.

Avoid animal proteins such as meats of all kinds, eggs, dairy; sugar in all its forms, bread, wheat pasta, white rice.

2. Hydrate

We are 80% water, and we lose 2L a day that are essential to replenish. Slight dehydration slows metabolism by 3%, and water loss by 3% decreases muscle strength and endurance by 10%, as well as physical and mental performance.

It is recommended to drink alkaline water. The formula to know how much water to drink is to multiply your weight by .033, and thus you will know how many liters exactly your body needs.

3. Emotional balance

Motivation is the basis for recovering our health, motivating ourselves in the way of eating, drinking and thinking, maintaining an alkaline diet is a lifestyle and although you may not believe it, negative thoughts or emotions cause stress, which generates more of acid in the body, that is why you must work in all aspects so you will maintain an emotional balance avoiding the lack of energy.

4. Re-mineralize

The body uses its mineral resources, such as sodium, potassium, calcium, and magnesium, to keep its alkaline design in balance. The acidity generated by the metabolism and the acidifying lifestyle consume the reserves that we must replace to preserve the optimal functioning of the organism.

You need minerals because:

- Minerals promote electrical conductivity, nerve impulses, and contraction of muscle fibers.
- The "sodium/potassium pump" allows information and nutrients to enter the cell.
- The treated "table" salt dehydrates and acidifies; therefore it can promote hypertension (99% sodium chloride)
- Sea and Himalayan salt do not promote hypertension.

When you don't have enough alkalizing minerals, your kidneys become overloaded; It is important to consume foods such as asparagus, beets, celery, and spinach.

5. Detoxify

Both metabolism and lifestyle (including diet) generate an accumulation of toxic acids in the body. There are several options to help you eliminate toxins:

- Fasting or semi-fasting
- Cold pressing purifying juices (detox plan)
- Liver and kidney cleansing
- Cleaning through colon hydrotherapy
- Cleansing through enemas